The LI

Success

Discover how to use LINCOMYCIN for the treatment of

severe bacterial and skin infection

Hess John

CHAPTER 1................... **Error! Bookmark not defined.**

LINCOMYCIN 6

SIDE EFFECTS OF THIS MEDICATION 7

LINCOMYCIN HYDROCHLORIDE 10

CHAPTER 2.. 12

INDICATIONS 12

DOSAGE AND ADMINISTRATION 13

DRUG INTERACTION 14

PRECAUTIONS 14

CHAPTER 3.. 16

LABORATORY TEST 16

PREGNANCY 16

NURSING MOTHERS 17

IN CHILDREN 17

WHAT TO KNOW ABOUT THIS MEDICATION .. 18

CHAPTER 4 20

HOW TO TAKE THIS MEDICATION 20

AT MISSED DOSE 21

AT OVERDOSE 21

WHAT TO AVOID 22

OTHER MEDICATION THAT AFFECTS THIS

DRUG 23

ACKNOWLEDGEMENT 25

CHAPTER 1

LINCOMYCIN

This medication is known to be a prescription medication used for the treatment of bacterial infection which is severe and also a good antibiotic for those who is allergic to penicillin antibiotics.

This drug can be administered on its own or alongside with other medication, it belongs to drug class known as antibiotics.

More research is needed to ascertain if this medication is safe to use in children younger than 1 month of age.

Also, this medication cannot be used for the treatment of

common cold, viral infections or flu.

SIDE EFFECTS OF THIS MEDICATION

This medication has the following side effects:

Chill

Cold

Fever

Tiredness

Skin sores

Severe diarrhea

Stomach pain

Breath shortness

Pale skin

Bloody stool

Cold hand and feet

Lightheadedness

Mouth ulcer

Inadequate urination

Mouth blisters

Severe bleeding

Swollen gum

Difficulty in swallowing

Jaundice

Try to speak to your health care professional should any

of the above side effects is noticed.

This medication has the most common side effects which are:

Dizziness

Diarrhea

Nausea

Stomach pain

Vomiting

Rash

Itching

Ringing in the ear

Swollen tongue

Painful tongue

Vagina discharge or itching

Try to speak to your health care professional should any of the above side effects is noticed or fails to go away after a while

This medication should only be administered in treating or preventing infections that has been suspected or proven to be caused by bacterial.

LINCOMYCIN HYDROCHLORIDE

Its hydrochloride form is known to be a white crystalline odorless powder. It has an acidic solution and is dextrorotatory. This form of lincomycin is freely soluble in water and other chemical solutions, but slightly soluble

in acetone.

CHAPTER 2

INDICATIONS

This medication is indicated in the treatment of the following:

Infections due to susceptible strains of streptococci

It is indicated for those that are allergic to penicillin antibiotics

Also, before this medication can be administered, one should have performed surgical procedures in conjunction with antibacterial therapy.

This medication (Lincomycin) can be administered alongside with other antimicrobial medication when indicated.

DOSAGE AND ADMINISTRATION

Should you have severe diarrhea while using this medication, discontinue it as soon as possible.

Intramuscular

Adult dose: 600mg every 24 hours

Severe infection: 600mg every 12 hours

Intravenous

Adult dose: 1g should be administered every 8 to 12 hours

Severe situation: 8g has been administered in life

threatening cases

NOTE: if more than the required dosage of this medication is administered, severe cardiopulmonary reaction may occur.

DRUG INTERACTION

This medication should be used cautiously in patient having or receiving neuromuscular blocking agents. This is because this medication has neuromuscular blocking properties.

PRECAUTIONS

Precautions should be taking in patients with the

following medical conditions:

Patient with colitis

Patient with gastrointestinal disease

Asthma patient

Patient that get allergic reactions easily

It should be administered cautiously in patient with pre-existing candida infections, if used, anti-fungal medication should be given alongside

This medication should be cautiously used in patient with renal or hepatic dysfunction

CHAPTER 3

LABORATORY TEST

If this medication has been administered for long, periodic liver and kidney function tests and blood counts should be carried out.

PREGNANCY

This medication should be avoided in pregnant individual, no adequate result or experiment has been conducted as regards this.

NURSING MOTHERS

This medication has been reported to appear I human milk. So as a nursing mother, discuss with your medical personnel to know if you are to put an end to this medication or discontinue nursing, your doctor will tell you what to do based on the discussion you both have.

IN CHILDREN

This medication causes Gasping syndrome in premature infants. The use of this medication I infant below the age of 1 month has not been established.

WHAT TO KNOW ABOUT THIS MEDICATION

Make sure you are not treated with this medication if you are allergic to it or its derivatives

Also, explain to your medical health personnel before taking this medication, most especially, those with the history of intestinal disorder such as:

Ulcerative colitis

You can as well let your health care professional be informed if you ever had the following:

Liver disease

Kidney disease

Asthma

Severe allergies

Asthma

Make sure you inform your medical health personnel if you are pregnant before you take this medication, it is not known if these medications harm an unborn baby.

CHAPTER 4

HOW TO TAKE THIS MEDICATION

This medication should be administered as directed, it should be used or taken with full glass cup of water.

This medication should be orally taken usually once daily or twice daily in severe cases. Take this medication with lots of water unless your doctor asked you no to do so.

The dosage of this medication is usually based on your condition and the response to your therapy

This antibiotic should as well be taken at evenly spaced time for proper effectiveness. It can be taken at same time daily to help you keep to the usual time. Keep up with your medication till you finish your prescribed amount or dosage, even if symptoms goes off, do not stop the use of this medication, stopping it may lead to relapse of the infection.

AT MISSED DOSE

Should you miss a dose, take it as soon as you remember, skip the missed dose should it's close to the time of the next dose. Do not take two dosses at a time to compliment the missed dose.

AT OVERDOSE

You can call poison help line or better still seek

emergency medical attention. Overdose symptoms include the following:

Seizures

Severe vomiting

Diarrhea that is persistent

Changes in amount of urine

WHAT TO AVOID

Most antibiotic medication causes diarrhea, and as such, showing a sign of new infection. Should you have a bloody or watery diarrhea, make sure you tell your health care professional before the use of any anti-diarrhea medication.

OTHER MEDICATION THAT AFFECTS THIS DRUG

Some other drugs that affect this medication are:

Vitamins

Prescription medications

Vitamins

Herbal medications

Make sure you talk to your health care professional about the drug you take presently, if you can stop the use, or continue its use with ampicillin

ABOUT THE AUTHOR

The author of this book named **Hess John** is a medical doctor and a notable writer of our time, he uses individualized knowledge to put down this basic guide.

ACKNOWLEDGEMENT

Glory to God for this success of this project, kudos to family and friends, you are all the best.

Made in United States
Troutdale, OR
12/15/2023